Alzheimer's

Catching Up With
The New Reality

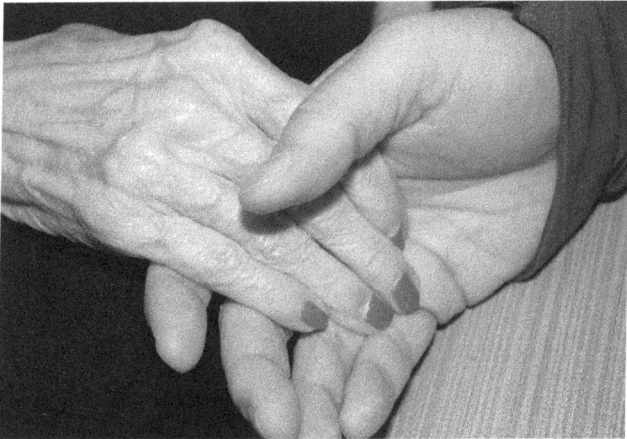

DAVID MAJOR

ISBN 10: 0-9655533-3-7
ISBN 13: 978-0-9655533-3-9

Edited by Victor Rook
Cover and Interior Design by Victor Rook

Cover Photo by David Major

Dedicated to my wife, Dale, who came into my life at the right moment and became a relentless caregiver to my Mom, Mike, and me. I couldn't have made it through this without you.

FOREWORD

I once heard that if you've seen one case of Alzheimer's, you've seen one case of Alzheimer's. No two are alike. But there are similarities, especially for the caregiver.

Being a caregiver is hard, heartbreaking, and ever changing. As your loved one goes through the stages of decline, each change puts you into a new reality of different circumstances.

I was reactive, never proactive. I never knew what was coming next. I wish I had this book to read before facing what I went through. This is one true story about my Mom and her battle with Alzheimer's from beginning to the very end.

PART ONE:

IN THE BEGINNING...

May 17, 2011 - Noticing a change

I stopped by to see my Mom and her husband, Mike. It was one of those perfunctory "check it off the list" tasks to keep a clear conscience that I am a good son. At the time, I was more interested in my own life. Of course, I would get the "you don't visit often enough" and "you don't stay long enough" responses to my visit.

They had both lost their spouses ten years prior, then met at church, and married about five years later. On the day of my visit they were both 81 years old. They were sitting at a table in the kitchen. The kitchen wasn't big enough for a table, but they had it in there anyway. It is where they read the paper, drank their coffee, and sat and talked. It was more sunny and comfortable than the formal dining room. Mom got up to fix me some coffee and fuss around with dishes. Mike kept reading the paper, so I sat down in her seat. I looked down and noticed the two medicine organizers. There were four compartments for each day: Morning, Lunch, Dinner, and Bedtime. It was a Tuesday, but Mom's organizer still had a pill in the Monday Lunch slot. Also, the pills for Wednesday Dinner were missing. I asked Mike about it. He was the one that ordered meds and put them in the organizers. He looked over from his paper unconcerned and said, "Sometimes she forgets to take her pills."

I wasn't all that fond of Mike in the first place, but not taking care of my mother was a stab in my heart. That moment is permanently etched in my brain. And it almost didn't happen, because I'm not the type to notice what's in a pillbox. Here's the thing: the first signs of Alzheimer's don't come at you in neon lights. It's subtle. You haven't experienced it so you don't know what to look for. And they aren't helping, either. They hide their increasing challenges to care for themselves. They don't want you to know. They want to stay at home and not be dragged off to a nursing home. Sure, they left the oven on that one time. Who hasn't? Mike gave up on his cherished garden. "Too much work." Mom didn't go to church as much because she couldn't remember people's names. Okay, that's different. No, the signs come at the edges of your peripheral vision. I almost missed noticing that missing pill.

Tip #1: They will hide their increasing disability.

Tip #2: The initial signs will be barely noticeable.

Mike knew the doctor's number by heart. I wrote it down. The next day I called. You have to leave a message, and you need the DOB (date of birth). Called Mom back and got her DOB. Called and left a message for the doctor. The nurse called back: they can't talk to me. As will happen many times in this journey, you will run into legal roadblocks. Got the forms for Mom and Mike to sign to give the doctor permission to talk to me. Got their signatures. Sent the forms in. Called and made an appointment with the doctor. Reason: a pill still in the Monday lunch slot.

June 7, 2011 - A Very Good Doctor

There were so many times we got lucky. One example was the care of a very good doctor. I took Mom and Mike for the appointment and he talked to each of them long enough to determine their conditions. He had known them for years and could see their decline. He would ultimately diagnose Mom with Alzheimer's and Mike with dementia. He ordered an In-Home visit by a registered nurse to survey their home environment.

June 20, 2011 - A Very Good Nurse

We lucked out again; a very smart nurse came to see them. Sandy was intelligent, vivacious, outspoken, and professional. The first thing she did was work with the doctor to simplify the meds. Instead of having to take meds four or five times a day, she got it down to just morning meds and evening meds. That helped a great deal. The next thing she did was "strongly suggest" that I take over ordering the meds, loading the pillboxes, and making sure they took them correctly. Sometimes it takes a baseball bat to get my attention, and this was a real wakeup call. She impressed upon me the need to take a more active role in their care.

My care for Mom would last 4 years, 7 months, and 17 days. Fortunately, I didn't know that. It wasn't a long time, not near as long as it could have been. And, fortunately, I had the time to give when it was needed the most. I remodel kitchens for a living and the poor economy had all but put me out of business.

June 22, 2011 - Looking For Help

So the first thing I did was go on online and look for information. I found and called Alzheimer's Association. It is a valuable resource, but unfortunately I didn't know what I needed. I must have expected them to send someone out to comfort me and take care of Mom and Mike. Of course, that didn't happen.

I called their church and talked to the secretary. Mom and Mike had been members for a long time and Mike was a deacon. She took my name and number to give to the preacher. He didn't return my call. A few weeks later I tried again. He never called back. No one from the church reached out.

I did find a really sweet lady that agreed to sit with Mom and Mike in the morning. Her job was to make sure they took their meds, ran any errands needed, and helped Mom with housework. The lady mostly just sat with them. Her low pay and low hours never amounted to much, but it still ruffled Mike to write the checks. The nice lady eventually quit, telling me that Mom and Mike needed more care than she could give them.

I talked to Mom and Mike about moving, but they didn't want to discuss it. My brother and sister questioned their safety. I agreed that Mom and Mike might burn the house down, or hurt themselves or others. Mike was still driving. But I also felt, and still do, that each day they could stay at home was incredibly precious. Their eventual move would prove to bring down their standard of living, their contentment, and their sense of freedom.

Meanwhile, Mom and Mike loved Whopper JRs from Burger King. I knew they liked to go there a lot. What I didn't know is that they went there every day, and sometimes twice a day. I didn't know they weren't cooking, and that the food in the pantry was years expired. I would have known that if I had looked. But I didn't think to do so.

On several occasions I got a call from the manager at Burger King. Mike had Gastroesophageal Reflux Disease (GERD) and it sometimes caused him to belch up his food. Each time I got there the mess had been cleaned up. The manager was always nice about it. And Mike would claim he was fine. He said he was fine every time, about everything.

One day Mom confided in me that Mike took the riding mower to the shop for servicing, but when they went back to pick it up, he couldn't find the shop. I picked up the mower and brought it to them. You would think that with all these incidents going on I would have wised up to the need for action.

I finally started to see Mom's decline. She could carry on a conversation but couldn't find all the words. It frustrated her. She feared Alzheimer's but wasn't suffering any of the middle stages of decline. Her personality had not changed, she wasn't too confused, and she could still dress herself and take care of household chores.

Tip #3: Your loved ones will move in and out of the Stages of Decline.

October 10, 2011 - More luck kicks in

Dale, my future wife, and I found each other on Match.com and met at a Panera Bread for coffee. Attraction was mutual and date nerves subsided right away. Best first date EVER. My phone rang. I looked at the number but didn't answer. I was way more interested in Dale. We got a second cup of coffee and continued to talk. Then that phone number flashed in my head: it was the number for the hospital. The reason I knew that number was because it periodically popped up when Mike was admitted into the ER. It was never anything life threatening. Frankly, I think Mike liked the hospital. He could stay in bed, watch TV, and get served his meals. Mom had retired from the phone company and her benefits were great, so coverage wasn't an issue.

I explained to Dale that I had to go to the hospital—it was right down the road—and asked if she would like to go with me. She said yes. She came along and we found Mom and Mike in the ER. After I introduced Dale to them, she went over to the bed, touched Mike on his knee, and asked how he was doing. As if I didn't know by then, I knew from that gesture that she was special. A true caregiver has the natural gift of the most powerful form of healing: touch. That day Dale came into my life, and she would eventually take over the lion's share of Mom and Mike's care.

October 17, 2011 - Looking at Retirement Homes

Dale went with me to look at retirement homes. The one we liked the best was called Golden Terrace. It was strategically located between my brother, my sister, and me. The rooms had a homey feel. There was a bedroom, bathroom, and an open area that included a kitchenette. A washer and dryer were down the hall. The facility had three floors on one side and three on the other. In the middle was the dining area. It was open to the top of the third floor, so it was bright and cheerful. They served three meals a day. Each round table could seat four. The chairs were big and comfortable, and seating was not assigned. Three meals a day, maid service, and no yard to mow— what's not the love? It was also very affordable.

So, how would we get them to move? I had heard horror stories of elderly people kicking and screaming as they were dragged out of their homes. I also knew people that moved themselves into a retirement home. But I don't think it is anyone's first choice. It was not Mom and Mike's intention, and it was their decision to make. I asked them to at least visit the place, but they refused.

December 14, 2011 - More luck kicks in

Mike needed a knee replacement and the procedure was scheduled for December 14. I took them to the hospital and got Mike admitted. Then I sat with Mom as we waited for Mike to come out of the operating room. Mom was mildly confused, so we couldn't leave her at home. Mike stayed in the hospital for five days. Mom sat with Mike all day, and I stayed in the Hospitality Room. Then I took her home in the evening. My sister stayed with her overnight. During those five days I picked up Mom in the morning and took her to go and sit with Mike. Each day that I stayed at the hospital, I brought a Harry Potter book. I had read them before, but enjoyed them all again.

The other patients on the floor were walking up and down the halls and recovering from their knee replacements. Mike didn't like to walk, he didn't like physical therapy, and so he wasn't recovering as well as the others. It dropped him down a notch mentally. As we would experience over and over, any change had a negative impact on them. It could be a surgical procedure, a move, or a fall.

Medical coverage for the hospital stay ended after five days, but he still couldn't walk. The hospital administrator arranged for him to be moved to an assisted-living facility to continue his physical therapy. She also arranged for his transportation and to have his prescriptions go with him.

The next morning I went to check on Mike at the new place, and I was appalled. Patients were two to a very small room. There was no privacy and not enough space for a chair next to his bed. The guy in the other bed was making use of the call button but was mostly ignored. Staff members were out in the hall in small groups carrying on with animated conversations. They seemed more interested in swapping stories than bothering with health care. I was livid.

Mike was groggy and disoriented. I found the supervisor and looked over his list of medications. They had gone down the list and given him all his meds, including Lunesta. How much brainpower does it take to know NOT to give him a sleeping pill in the morning? The supervisor's response was vague and defensive. I sensed that she was experienced at covering for mistakes. I went back to Mike and promised that I would get him out of there. He nodded, but I don't think he understood me.

Meanwhile, the office manager at Golden Terrace made me an offer I couldn't refuse. He would give me the rest of December rent-free and pay to move in their furniture. I signed up and called my brother and sister to help with the move. Two days later we had Mom and Mike moved into a cozy, one-bedroom apartment. It had a living area with a kitchenette, a bathroom, and a bedroom large enough for their king-size bed. There was room for their kitchen table, and that was important to me. We found Mom's ceramic Christmas tree and some decorations, which were pretty dismal, actually. Fortunately, Golden Terrace had amazing Christmas decorations throughout the facility.

We told Mike that he was there (under doctor's orders) for physical therapy, which was right down the hall. We alluded that it was probably temporary (not). In the meantime, he could wheel himself down to meals three times a day.

And that is how we got Mom and Mike from their home to a retirement home. He kinda did it to himself.

January 1, 2012 - First check to Golden Terrace: $3,050

Not a bad deal for rent, utilities, cable, and three meals a day.

January 4, 2012 - The doctor signs Mom's and Mike's Power of Attorney documents

Years before, Mom and Mike had planned for the future. They had wills drawn up. A prenuptial agreement kept Mom's real estate and investments in a trust that would be inherited by her children. If she died first, Mike would have lifetime rights to live in the house, but it would stay in her trust. I was named trustee. Mom had a Power of Attorney document that gave my sister POA upon signature of the doctor that she was no longer capable of caring for herself. Mike had a POA document that gave my brother POA upon signature of the doctor. He signed them on January 4, 2012. Why would Mike give my brother this authority and responsibility instead of his own daughter? Let's just say there was a trust issue there.

I can't imagine the anguish Mike must have experienced to lose his independence, freedom, and control. He was quiet and amiable but fiercely proud. He was a member of our Greatest Generation. He grew up in the backwoods of Maine and made it through the 8th grade, but then he needed to work on the farm full time. At 18 he joined the Army and served in WWII and then another tour in Korea. He married and worked as a bus driver for 35 years. After his wife died, he met my Mom and they married a few years later. It was probably the easiest years of his life. Mom had the house paid for, full medical coverage, a good pension, and social security. So his pension and social security were mostly his to spend as he wished. As a product of his generation, he was the man of the house and king of his castle. I'm sure it was devastating to lose his kingdom.

Mom was also a member of the Greatest Generation and treated Mike as head of the household. However, she did try to persuade him to have better manners, flush the toilet, and stop farting in public.

The nice thing about having the Physical Therapists (PT) people in-house was that I could get them to check that Mom and Mike took their morning meds. This favor was not in the PT's job description, but they were very nice about helping out. Evening meds were still my responsibility, as were weekend meds and ordering meds.

March 2012 - Vodka steps in as a caregiver's crutch

Caregiving is stressful. It is hard. It is heartbreaking to slowly lose someone to dementia. The caregiver is totally helpless to do anything to stop the inevitable. My evenings were permanently reserved for dispensing meds. And checking Mike's blood-sugar level.

Another task was to load the coffee maker. They loved morning coffee. So I found one with a timer so I could get it ready the night before. They also liked Little Debbie snack cakes, so we kept them on hand.

But it was sad. Unrewarding. Relentless. After my tasks were completed, I would say goodnight and leave. In less than one year they changed from my parents to my children. It was like leaving eight-year-olds to fend for themselves. This was the worst stage of Alzheimer's because they were most aware of losing their freedom. They always wanted me to stay. Their room was on the second floor at the far end. There was a door right across the hall from their room that led to steps to the parking lot. I could barely make it through that door before my eyes started watering. By the time I got to the first floor, I was crying buckets.

My choice of self-medication was White Russians. Plural. With pretzels. While watching recorded golf tournaments, which is sort of like watching grass grow. The buzz helped soften the pain. But, among other things, vodka is fattening. One day I stepped on the scale, looked at the number, and kicked the scale across the room. Then I hopped around on one foot while yelling, and I walked with a limp the rest of the day. I stopped drinking because it was making me fat.

My point is to warn not to neglect the caregiver. Care for *you* first. Put on your mask first. Pamper yourself. You are the other victim. Put yourself in the shoes of your best friend and give yourself his or her advice. Then take the advice. Don't be a martyr. Seek help. Hire help. Try not to let it pull you down. And above all, forgive yourself for what you can't do. You can't do it all.

Tip #4: Don't let their illness harm you.

Hate the disease not the person

One of the symptoms of dementia is a change of personality. They start to lose their social filters. Mom and Mike threw out some insults, but at least we knew what was on their mind. So their core personality didn't really change much, but getting them to remember something was frustrating. I recall my brother admonishing Mom one day: "Mom! Don't forget to take your meds tomorrow morning!" Mom nodded obediently, but her eyes were blank. She would not remember, no matter how often we repeated ourselves. Communication was on a much lower level, if at all.

It is up to you to adapt to the changes. You will deal less and less with the person and more and more with the disease.

Tip #5: Communication will change and decline.

So where is God?

Mom and Mike worked all their lives, "doing unto others," and not hurting anyone. So why the punishment of dementia? Why can't we just die in our sleep? I'm okay with death. If life were too long it wouldn't be precious.

I also understand that it takes more than old age to kill us. At our primordial core is the instinct to survive and procreate. Our skin can repair cuts. We can develop resistance to infections. If hypothermic, our brain cuts off blood supply to extremities to keep the core warm. Our heartbeat and breathing increase to face a fight or flight confrontation. And all of this is done without conscious thought. We are built to prevail. So it takes something like dementia or cancer to kill us. But why a long, painful process? Why the heartache of the victim and the family, and the effort it takes?

At first I decided not to believe in God. No God worth my worship would be so cruel. But then I decided I couldn't be mad at Him if I wasn't a believer. Then I decided I was a believer and pissed. Then I thought it probably wasn't a good idea to be mad at God. Still, how could there be a

God and a disease that ate your brain? Ultimately, I decided that I do believe in something. I believe a lingering death sucks.

May 2012 - Mike's daughter shows up with another nail for their coffin.

Her name is Judy and her last name starts with "F." My sister's name is also Judy, so we started calling Mike's daughter Judy F. She came into town and bought plane tickets for Mom and Mike to go to Maine to visit his family. Judy F is very aggressive and pushy and everything is fast-forward, except thinking. I wanted to confront her, but I was up against both her and Mike. Backing down, I did have to admit that the trips to Maine were a highlight of their lives. For Mike, of course, but even for Mom. His brothers and sisters and their families loved Mom and how much she meant to their brother.

Pro: It would be their last vacation. They would enjoy the trip. I would be free from May 11 to May 25, 2011.

Con: If it didn't kill them, it would certainly pull them down another notch, and the notch down would be permanent.

I loaded their meds and called ahead to give instructions. Mostly I spoke with the wife of one of Mike's brothers. She could speak openly and I learned that Mom and Mike were welcome, but not Judy F.

Judy F picked them up and took them to the airport. I called and asked her for the airline and flight number and she responded that Mom and Mike left at Gate 6. She didn't remember the airline and didn't know anything about a flight number. But they left at Gate 6.

They got to Maine okay and all was well for a few days. Then a call came with a question: "Did you know Mike is incontinent?" Well, he could be a little gamey sometimes.

I was embarrassed that I was constantly catching up to the next level of decline. I was never prepared for the next problem. Never had a clue what was coming next.

Up in Maine, they bought diapers and cleaned up after Mike. They reported that for the most part he just wanted to lie down and spent little time socializing. They said Mom was sweet but obviously confused. At the end of the visit Mom and Mike were put on the plane, with explanation of their condition. They missed their connection but were put up in a hotel. The airline picked them up the next morning and brought them to the airport. And they got them on the plane. Mom and Mike got back and seemed five years older. I felt guilty that I let Judy F mistreat them.

Tip #6: Don't let well-meaning relatives do harm.

July 2012 - The cavalry arrives (cue bugle music)

Dale and I had been dating since the previous fall. She had been helping with many of the responsibilities, sometimes without me. But in July our relationship got to the next level and she moved in with me. She set about the tasks of turning my house into a home. And she took over the care of Mom and Mike. She took them to Burger King. She showered them. She did their laundry. She cleaned the bathroom to her approval. And she took charge of Mike. Dale's background was working as a Nurse Assistant at the Veterans Hospital. So she knew how to handle cantankerous old men.

Mike didn't like to take showers. He sometimes refused to take showers. Dale made him take showers, most of the time. Sometimes his stubbornness won out.

Golden Terrace had rocking chairs out the front door and under a canopy. Mom and Mike liked to go out there and rock. But sometimes Dale would find Mom by herself because Mike had gone upstairs to take a nap. They kept missing meals because they didn't know the time. They didn't know the time of day and couldn't remember what time meals were served. My sister found a large, bright display board that showed the month, time, day, year, date, and day of the week. I loved it and looked at it often. I don't think Mom and Mike ever did.

7/27/2012 - Dale finds Mom wandering in the hall looking for the bathroom. She is wearing two bras and three shirts. Mike is nowhere around.

It's time to rent the house

Back when Mom and Mike were still living in the house, Judy F showed up to take "what her Daddy wanted her to have." Most of his stuff was junk and good riddance, but there was a rub that, excuse me, they're not dead yet. Judy F literally backed up a trailer to the front door. She also wanted the riding mower, the one we used to mow the large lawn with. Her Daddy wanted her to have it, but I found a lock in my truck and put it on the door to the shed. She was spitting mad, but she had to leave without it.

After Mom and Mike moved into Golden Terrace, we started to empty the house. I figured it would take three trips: one with my family to come and claim what they wanted, a day for a yard sale, and a day to take all the rest of the stuff to Goodwill. It took months and months.

First, nobody wanted anything. No one needed another dining room table, chairs, and hutch. No one wanted an entertainment center, sofa, end tables, and lamps. No one wanted knick-knacks.

My brother, Mark, and my sister, Judy, took over the task of pricing everything for a yard sale. It took them weeks to do, in between their heavy work schedules. The first yard sale cleared a lot, but left a lot, too. The next yard sale cleared more. Part of the problem was that we kept setting things aside because we couldn't decide if we could let them go. Eventually, it just became a chore to get stuff out. Then more chores to clean the place. That is when we found the outdated cans of food.

Then we discovered that the heat pump needed servicing, some of the rooms needed painting, and the bathroom needed updating. We all pitched in and got it done. We rented it to two Asian gentlemen that had transferred to Richmond to follow their jobs. They were programmers. Their English was poor. We never told Mom and Mike the house was rented.

8/27/2012 - We took Mom to the doctor. She had a Urinary Tract Infection (UTI). We would eventually learn that when Mom got mean and cussed, she had a UTI. I was actually a little bit amused when she got that way. I had never known her as anything but polished and proper.

8/29/2012 - Mike got mad at me that twenty percent of his money wasn't going to the church. I was respectful of everything I could regarding his wants and wishes. But I was not about to send money to the people that forgot about him. Also, I remembered a comment my Mom made. It was on one of the trips home from visiting Mike at the hospital after his knee surgery. We passed their church and she pointed out the new roof. Then she expressed her disagreement with Mike for giving so much to the church. "We probably financed that roof," she said, frowning.

I also stopped the lawn service. I cancelled Orkin. There were daily requests in the mail requesting more contributions. Noble cause or not I ignored them. His money would hence go toward his and my Mom's care.

I read that elderly dementia victims are vulnerable to solicitors. That might be true, but I think that for Mike it was his pride and pleasure to be able to give. I think disposable income was new to him. Years before he received a very nice knife from one of the charities he supported. I commented that he must have given them a lot to get a knife that nice as a thank you. His reply was that he liked to "give his fair share."

Tip #7: Early on, get in their business. Be nosey. Protect them from solicitors.

9/3/2012 - **Mom wanders out and down the street**

A majority of wandering Alzheimer's victims seek woods or water. Mom headed to both. To the west was a creek and it was in a wooded area. Interestingly, her home was in the opposite direction. As usual, I did not see that coming. The call came from the police. A lady found Mom walking down the street early in the morning. She called the police and they figured out where Mom came from. Mom was safe, but it scared us.

Technology could have helped. We needed to know if Mom's physical location changed from about midnight to eight the next morning. Or if their door opened. We would probably need help from the staff.

I immediately began looking for Assisted Living. In the meantime, something had to be done about Mom wandering again. Golden Terrace didn't have any form of restricted access. If someone walked up to the front door from the inside, the sliding doors would part, day or night. So we took turns getting up and driving over to guard the front door. The doors didn't open going in until 7 AM. So we sat in the parking lot until we could go in and confirm that Mom was still there. We did that every morning, until we decided on an assisted-living facility.

PART TWO:

A COLLECTION OF HEARTACHES

9/17/2012 - We move Mom and Mike to Assisted Living

Once you leave the normal environment of a retirement home, you enter the heartless world of elderly care. I will refer to the facility as the Institute of Indifference (IOI). My first shock was that their facility might not be able to take Mike in the Memory Care Unit. It was on the second floor and had restricted access. Mom had Alzheimer's, Mike had dementia. The Director of Nursing suggested that Mike might do better down on the first floor. *Whaaat?* It boggles my mind that people in health care think it might be a good idea to separate a married couple. Splitting up a married couple doesn't even sound legal, much less moral. Other than providing comfort for each other, what did they have to live for? The good doctor came to our rescue again and signed off on papers that "proved" Mike's inability to care for himself. And that "qualified" him to stay with his wife. Roadblock avoided.

I took all of Mom's and Mike's medicines to the IOI. The Director of Nursing (I will call her DON) informed me that the meds would have to be blister packed, and there would be a charge. They would start using their pharmacy, not my insurance-supported pharmacy. I had to agree that blister packs helped keep the meds straight. You wouldn't want a Monday pill still there on Tuesday. And I was free of ordering, organizing, and dispensing meds. Yay!

Tip #8: Assisted Living facilities are licensed by the State Department of Social Services. So, Assisted Living facilities report to the government, not to residents.

I knew the move would knock Mom and Mike down another notch. We contracted a turnkey mover to move everything, including pictures on the walls. It needed to be as seamless as possible. My sister (Judy, no F) drove Mom and Mike to the IOI. She took them to the courtyard and sat in the gazebo. My brother, Mark, and I worked with the movers. The new home had a small bedroom, a bathroom, and a fair-sized living area. Their dresser wouldn't fit in the bedroom so it went into the living area. Mike would have his recliner, and Mom would have her upholstered chair.

More luck, there must be a God!

There was a lead CNA (Certified Nurse Assistant) on the second floor and her name was Delores. Delores was an angel from heaven. She walked up to Mom (now Miss Jane) and took her by the hand. She took Mom around the courtyard, always holding her. I have to think about it to remember if Delores was big or small, white or black. Instead, what pops up first is her voice talking to Mom and saying, "Miss Jane, I love you."

Delores also took charge of Mike and was one of only a few people that could get him to take a shower. She made sure he got his paper and knew how he liked his coffee.

Compared to the location of Golden Terrace, the IOI was closer to Dale and I, about the same to Judy, and farther for Mark. It would have been better to have a place centrally located, but that didn't happen. It was 1.8 miles from my house and took about five minutes to get there. On several occasions there were emergencies and it took us less than two minutes to get there.

Tip # 9: Location, location, location. Keep them close.

One of the services was laundry, and clothes started disappearing immediately. So Dale took over the laundry. That meant bringing it home, and Mike's clothes were pretty rank. Sometimes his penis would pop out of the diaper and he would pee down his leg. We could wash the socks, but sometimes we would have to just buy new shoes.

Dale is a small woman, about size 2. Toting the laundry around was hard on her, and I didn't know it. She didn't complain and I didn't notice. I regret that.

Tip # 10: Don't be stupid like me.

Mom and Mike were the new kids on the block, and that was unfortunate. Not only were the other residents scary, but Mom and Mike were cognitive enough to know it. Especially for Mom, who did not want to live in a dorm. She and Mike sat off to themselves as much as possible. We would learn that every time a new resident came in, they would want to go home.

Alzheimer's victims move in and out of the stages of decline. Some days are better than others, and those days give hope. But good days are outnumbered by bad days, and over a period of time there is decline. Even on any given day, they can be cognitive in the morning and then "sundown" in the evening. They become more agitated, irritable, and confused as the day wears on.

The weather is an influence. Sunny days can perk them up and rainy days can bring them down. Their condition changes during a full moon. It can get crazy in the Memory Unit during that time. And when an infection runs through the floor, basically the wheels fall off the wagon. Illness on top of dementia is so cruel. Decline during an illness seems to be more permanent.

9/25/2012 - Dale reports one of Mom's comments: "Maybe when I die I will go to heaven and remember things again."

9/27/2012 - Mom randomly "packs" her clothes, moving them from drawer to drawer. At first we labeled the drawers. Why did we do that? Mom didn't read the labels, and if she did, she wouldn't remember.

10/14/2012 - Mom has chest pains. She is rushed to the ER. There is a lump in her left breast.

10/25/2012 - A biopsy is performed to determine if the lump is malignant. A mammogram is also done. Mom needed to hold still for the X-ray, so Dale stayed in the room and held her. They covered up Dale as much as possible, but she was still exposed to the radiation. No one liked the idea, but it needed to be done, and Dale insisted she be there.

10/30/2012 - Mike still had a phone and still knew the doctor's number. He called and made an appointment. I don't know why he did that. He didn't remember doing it later. The appointment was cancelled.

12/14/2012 - The lump in Mom's breast was malignant, so a mastectomy was performed. The procedure was done as outpatient.

January 2013

Mom weighs 126 lbs. Mike weighs 184 lbs.

1/8/2013 - Mom fell out of bed and hit the side of her head. She was taken to the ER and received four stitches. That afternoon she didn't remember that she had fallen. Mike didn't either. I bought a bed rail to catch up with this new problem. As usual, I was never getting ahead of a problem.

1/30/2013 - Mom gets a walker. Mike tries to put on Mom's sports bra as underwear. We are still taking them to Burger King now and then.

February 2013

Mom weighs 125 lbs. (down 1). Mike weighs 184 lbs. (no change)

2/20/2013 - Mom can't speak a whole sentence. She thought Dale was a high school friend.

2/28/2013 - Mike slides out of bed. What does it take for me to learn something? I JUST bought a bed rail for Mom. Why didn't I get two? So I bought one for Mike.

March 2013

Mom weighs 125 lbs. (no change). Mike weighs 184 lbs. (no change)

3/10/2013 - In the Memory Unit there are two groups at meals: those that can feed themselves, and those that can't. The ones that can't are referred to as "Feeders." There should be enough staffing to help all the Feeders, but that rarely happens. Mom got to where she couldn't feed herself, but we didn't want her in with the Feeders. So Dale started feeding Mom at lunch. It was the biggest meal.

By that time we knew the names of the other twenty or so residents. We had our favorites. Dale always gave Bonnie a hug and kidded with her that they were going to run away and join the circus. It never grew old and Bonnie always laughed.

We felt for the other residents. They rarely got visited. Some of them never got a visit. And most of them, or *all* of them, wanted to go home at some point.

One in particular stood next to the elevator and yelled at anyone that tried to keep her away. The staff couldn't physically move her, so it took a lot of consoling and redirection. On one occasion the staff person had to walk with me down to the other end of the building to get the elevator. With a different resident, we simply told her I was going up to the third floor, not down to the first floor. There was no third floor.

We knew most of the staff. Some were sweet, and some were just punching a time clock. Deloris was still there, but she was not always assigned to Mom and Mike. The staff was partly grateful for our presence, but partly wary of us as well. We knew stuff. We observed mistreatment. And we spoke up about it. From their website you would think that all is wonderful. Here is what it says:

Our residents' families are always welcome. We appreciate family involvement in our activities. We encourage families to visit regularly, and consider them a part of the staff. Together we can make our residents' stay a pleasant experience.

We didn't see much family involvement. And we were not made to feel like a part of the staff. For one thing, the staff thought they knew more about caring for the elderly than we did. They might have known more than me, but they didn't know more than Dale. So they didn't really appreciate being reminded to wash the residents' hands before meals. And then reminded again and again.

They didn't like it when I pointed out that staff was setting the temperature down to their comfort level. The staff was young and moving around, so they wanted it cooler. The elderly residents were sitting still and had slow metabolisms. They needed it warmer. Management agreed, but that didn't stop staff from setting the thermostat down to their liking. And they didn't bother to dress the residents warmer.

There were problems with the food. It was cold and tasteless. At first, plates were prepared downstairs with a lid put on, like at the hospital. But hospitals use insulated food carts. The IOI used push carts. So the food was cold. There was no butter for the rolls. There was no salt or pepper. Many times no coffee was brewed. Some meals, like chicken, needed to be cut, but the residents were too weak to cut it. Or they didn't have a knife. And staff didn't think to cut it for them beforehand. And yet, probably because of a requirement thought up by some detail-oriented, paranoid pencil-pusher, staff was required to log the percentage of the meal eaten for each resident and for each meal.

Eventually, after we complained constantly, the staff started using food carts. That was much better. The food arrived upstairs warm, and each plate was prepared one at a time. A new chef was hired and we started seeing gravy. And why not? The residents are not training for a marathon. Pile on the gravy. Pour in the sugar. Add salt, and pepper. And BUTTER. Lots of butter. Seriously, we are not trying to keep these people alive. We're trying to give them something to live for.

That's why most of my problem was with the DON. She was little about nursing and a whole lot about *administrivia*. In all fairness, there is probably a lot of paperwork for her to do. But there needed to be a supervisor of some sort. Someone to keep the staff accountable, informed, trained, and also happy. There was no one to do that. I took my complaints to the owner, but his response was that I might be happy somewhere else. Really, he said that.

I couldn't move Mom and Mike; each move bumped them down a notch and they were running out of notches. Time and again I tried to figure out a way to bring them home. I estimated $15/hour based on quotes I got for hired help for two people. I used 24 hours per day because I didn't think I could chance something happening to them at night—or them waking us up. So that came to $10,800/month before adding in food and other expenses.

I couldn't do it—not financially, not physically, and not emotionally. At the same time, I feel that the elderly should be kept at home and weaved into the fabric of our life. Our life should change so that the elderly are a natural part of the family. You should not drop off an elderly loved one like you drop the dog off at the kennel. Come to think of it, you shouldn't do that either. I am conflicted about this.

April 2013

Mom weighs 116 lbs. (down 9). Mike weighs 178 lbs. (down 6)

3/24/2013 - 4/2/2013 - Dale and I went on a vacation to Key Largo, Florida. Some of it was structured, some of it not. We had a great time, especially on the warm days. We hate the cold. Got back and the next day we visited Mom and Mike. We were shocked. They had lost a lot of weight in our absence. It made me feel guilty. We hadn't noticed the weight loss when visiting almost every day. The trip gave us perspective. That month, Mom lost 9 pounds and Mike lost 6 pounds. We started feeding Mom at dinners. Mark, Judy, and I took turns. Dale kept feeding her at lunch. We got their weights back up. I started a spreadsheet to track their weights. I asked the DON to give me their weights each month. I had to ask her each month.

4/21/2013 - Mom had a fall, but we didn't get a call. Dale noticed a bruise and asked about it. No one knew what had happened, but they found where it had been logged by the previous shift. After more prodding we learned that the shift log isn't available to the incoming shift. Instead, it is taken downstairs to be recorded. The log book returns back upstairs during the middle of the next shift. The DON doesn't interact with her staff, so each shift is clueless about what happened on the previous shift.

May 2013

Mom weighs 117 lbs. (up 1!).Mike weighs 174 lbs. (down 4)

5/3/2013 - Dale notices a new pill being given to Mom. "What's that?" she asked. "Antibiotic for UTI," was the tech's reply. And you were going to tell us about it when?

That same day Mom had a fall. It was probably related to the UTI. She was taken to the hospital. A bruise developed on her inner thigh.

5/14/2013 - Mom is lethargic. She reaches out to grab something in the air.

The reason I know about the dates is from Dale. Ever the professional caregiver, Dale was in the habit of keeping notes. She recorded each of the 26 times Mike had a fall, and the 9 times Mom had a fall. She even recorded the times we were not informed about a fall. She logged the times she asked the staff to wash the residents' hands before eating. She logged all the arguments with the DON. She lost track of Mom's UTIs.

Dale is a relentless caregiver. She is totally devoted to her children, grandchildren, sister, and in this case, my family and me. So she never let anything slide. The only reason she didn't bump heads with the DON more often is because the DON was rarely on the second floor.

Had it not been for Dale, I would have thought the IOI was doing their job. I would not have known to expect more, and been informed when things were wrong. I would have probably just come to visit, got bored quickly, then returned home. Had it not been for Dale, I would have had a lower sense of responsibility. I had to step up to her level of love.

Now I know that dropping your Mom off at the IOI is equivalent to boarding the dog. The "Pet Resort" will protect and feed your dog, and for a little extra money they will walk your dog once or twice or however much you pay for. The staff will be animal lovers, and they will do their best to provide a safe place for your pet—and still make a profit.

The IOI will feed and bath your loved one. And administer prescriptions. And check on them at least every two hours during the night. Which they do, according to some regulation, by first ringing the room's doorbell. It was probably instituted to keep staff from barging in. Maybe that was a problem. But the "fix" was a loud doorbell they rang every time they entered. It was always startling, and I never got used to it. Mom and Mike didn't like it either. I put some Band-Aids around where the plunger hit the chimes and that helped.

But the IOI will not love your loved one (except for Deloris). They are running a business and resources are stretched. In some cases, you wouldn't leave your dog where you put your loved one.

Tip # 11: The level of care given at a facility depends on you. You need to KNOW what is going on in there.

June 2013

Mom weighs 115 lbs. (down 2). Mike weighs 174 lbs. (no change)

6/15/2013 - Mom wants to go home. It was the most consistent thing she said throughout her different levels of decline. It stabbed my heart every time she said it. She also thought someone was going to kill her. I knew her belief was real to her. So I didn't say, "No, no one is trying to kill you." Instead I said, "Maybe so, but I am here and I will protect you." And then I would hold her.

July 2013

Mom weighs 112 lbs. (down 3). Mike weighs 174 lbs. (no change)

7/29/2013 - Mike fell in the doorway, tried to catch himself, and got his wedding ring caught on the latch. It broke his finger and the ring had to be cut off in the ER. The finger never healed right. Staff didn't try very hard to keep the bandages on or the splint in place. We later gave the ring to his daughter.

August 2013

Mom weighs 109 lbs. (down 3). Mike weighs 174 lbs. (no change)

8/1/2013 – We kicked out the tenants at Mom's house. They never missed a payment and did no harm to the property. But I make all my major decisions based on emotion (and it always works out). I stopped by and found the grass up to my knees. The tenants claimed the mower didn't work and they tried to fix it. And that they otherwise kept the grass cut. Then one of them pulled out his phone and showed me a picture taken in the front yard when the grass was cut.

"See?" he said. "We keep grass cut."

He was standing knee-deep in grass but thought reality was the picture in his phone.

It was an emotional decision. They had disgraced the memory of Mom's pride in her home. Mom would have never let her yard be an eyesore to her neighbors. The emotional sting for me was the combination of Mom wanting to come home and the home needing her to come back. I was livid and yelled at them to GET OUT.

8/6/2013 - Dale gives up doing the laundry. After 318 loads of wash, enough was enough. She had been doing the staff's job. Let them do it. We bought extra socks and underwear and towels to fill in for the lost laundry to come, which it did. On a few occasions we noted other residents wearing Mom's clothes. Dale's "extra" time was spent sitting with Mom.

Tip #12: Laundry WILL be lost. Buy extra clothes.

During that time Mark and Judy jumped in on preparing the house to sell. There was painting to do, some repairs, and removing yet more stuff. If there had been only one of us, it would have been impossible to accomplish what we did.

8/13/2013 – Dale got Mom a wheelchair. Using a walker was getting too dangerous. As designed today, all walkers are dangerous. It is difficult to walk in them correctly. You ALWAYS see a person bent over, arms outstretched, and pushing the walker in front of them. You are supposed to stand up straight. No one does. They need to be redesigned.

September 2013

Mom weighs 105 lbs. (down 4). Mike weighs 173 lbs. (down 1)

9/5/2013 - It is Mom's birthday. Dale bought and wrapped two scarves. One was red and the other was black and white stripes. It took a while for Mom to get the box unwrapped. There was surprise and pleasure on her face as she looked at her presents. She ran her hands over the fabric, lovingly. Then we had cake and ice cream. After cleaning up we put the box back on Mom's lap. She looked up at us in confusion, then down at the box. There was surprise and pleasure on her face as she looked at her scarves. She ran her hands over the fabric, lovingly. We never saw those scarves again.

October 2013

Mom weighs 114 lbs. (up 9!). Mike weighs 177 lbs. (up 4!)

10/26/2013 - Found Mike in Mom's wheelchair. He likes it better than using his walker, even though it is too small for him. And he likes being pushed in it.

10/27/2013 - Found Mike in Mom's wheelchair and Mom pushing him down the hall for lunch. I fussed at Mike about it, but words to him tended to vaporize after spoken.

At dinner, Mom cries. She wants to go back to Bluefield (where she grew up). That night I sent an email to my brother and sister. We sent emails to keep each other up to date. Home was now Bluefield, not Henrico County. It was the new reality. My sister came up with the phrase. One day she said, "You know, when there is a change with Mom or Mike it becomes the new set of circumstances we have to deal with. It becomes the new reality. So we deal with the new challenges." The phrase stuck and it seemed as if I was always catching up to the new reality. If only I had a crystal ball to tell me what was coming next.

November 2013

Mom weighs 118 lbs. (up 4). Mike weighs 175 lbs. (down 2)

11/1/2013 - Sold the house. Invested the proceeds, various levels of liquidity.

December 2013

Mom weighs 115 lbs. (down 3). Mike weighs 177 lbs. (up 2)

12/21/2013 - Winter Solstice: the shortest day and the longest night. Symbolic for me in that the days get longer from that day forward, bringing more light and more warmth. Dale and I married that day, and the future has been brighter ever since.

12/25/2013 - Wasn't that concerned about being there on Christmas Day. We had Christmas with Mom and Mike whenever we wanted. Several times a year we played and sang Christmas songs. Christmas Day itself was spent with the kids and grandkids.

January 2014

Mom weighs 117 lbs. (up 2). Mike weighs 176 lbs. (down 1)

February 2014

Mom weighs 121 lbs. (up 4). Mike weighs 172 lbs. (down 4)

March 2014

Mom weighs 124 lbs. (up 3). Mike weighs 169 lbs. (down 3)

PART THREE:

PROGRESSIVE SETS OF NEW REALITIES

3/20/2014 - Mom doesn't know who Dale is. This is the new reality now. I couldn't help but feel a little sting about that. But my day was coming.

It's Spring! Always a busy time. Between us, Dale and I have five kids and eight grandkids. Any given day could include a soccer game and a visit to Mom…and a cookout with one of the families…and having some grandkids over for the night. I do have a job, too, by the way. My lawn was rarely groomed and weeds ran amuck. There just wasn't the time.

We were lucky. We only cared for Mom and Mike. Members of the sandwich generation care for parents while still raising kids. The club sandwich generation is caring for parents, kids, and their kids. One of the problems is that we are living too long. Another problem is economics. Sometimes getting the kids out of the nest takes longer. According to one study, one in eight

Americans aged 40 to 60 is caring for a parent and raising a child.

In our case, we weren't raising kids or grandkids. It's just that the calendar stayed full. A blank date on the calendar created a vortex that sucked in an appointment or occasion.

April 2014

Mom weighs 124 lbs. (no change). Mike weighs 165 lbs. (down 4)

4/17/2014 - Mike thinks he is in New Jersey. Mom "packs" to take him home. Mike has no connection to New Jersey.

Every now and then someone expressed condolences regarding Mom. I replied that all was well. I had lost Mom long ago. The crying and mourning were over. Boy, was I wrong.

4/18/2014 - Sent an email to report a new reality. The note was short: "Today, Mom was fed by a stranger: Me."

So, basically, I lost her again. I cried on the way home.

May 2014

Mom weighs 125 lbs. (up 1). Mike weighs 165 lbs. (no change)

June 2014

Mom weighs 125 lbs. (no change). Mike weighs 157 lbs. (down 8)

July 2014

Mom weighs 125 lbs. (no change). Mike weighs 157 lbs. (no change)

7/14/2014 - Dale was still buying the pull-ups, shampoo, toothpaste, Ensure, Glucerna, etc. I don't know who else would have kept up with these things. The IOI didn't. I didn't know to buy these things, because I didn't know what I didn't know. Life would have been a lot different without Dale.

August 2014

Mom weighs 128 lbs. (up 3). Mike weighs 164 lbs. (up 7)

8/1/2014 - More help, this time from the Federal Government.

I received the first check from the Department of Veterans Affairs. It all began back in May of 2012 when we were still at Golden Terrace. I noticed a brochure about a local broker that would help with the application for Veteran Benefits—for free. At first I ignored it. I doubted anything good could come from the Federal Government. And I also doubted a local broker would do anything for free. But the staff at Golden Terrace said it was legitimate and I should look into it.

I met with the broker, and I was convinced it was for real because the paperwork was overwhelming. I needed Mike's birth certificate, marriage certificate to his first wife, her birth and death certificate, enlistment/discharge papers (from the 1940s, typed on a manual typewriter), forms signed by his doctor, and financial forms. I also needed Mom's birth certificate, marriage certificate to Dad, and Dad's birth and death certificates. It took me until 3/15/2013 to send in the application. It was approved 1/2/2014 for payments to begin on 4/1/2014. The payments accumulated until the processors could get the first check out on 8/1/2014. The extra money was a lifesaver. As Mom and Mike's care level increased, the cost went up as well. In the last few months, more money was going out than coming in.

September 2014

Mom weighs 128 lbs. (no change). Mike weighs 165 lbs. (up 1)

October 2014

Mom weighs 132 lbs. (up 4). Mike weighs 168 lbs. (up 3)

10/9/2014 - Mom wants to go home. Tells Dale: "Mike doesn't love me." "Don't look at me." "Don't touch me."

10/30/2014 - More comments to Dale: "I'm scared." "I'm afraid." "Who are you?"

Meanwhile, Mike reads his paper. I can't tell if he is *actually* reading it. Seems to take a long time. He eats well, and he likes to nap all afternoon.

November 2014

Mom weighs 133 lbs. (up 1). Mike weighs 169 lbs. (up 1)

11/14/2014 - Mom and Mike change to "mechanical soft" food. It's the new reality. As dementia patients decline they forget to chew. Or chew enough. They become a choking risk. Mechanical soft is not a bad thing. The chicken is ground up, for example. It's still meat and looks like meat. No celery or raw vegetables are allowed, though. Cooked vegetables are minced. Mashed potatoes are okay, and everything else is soft. The residents are fed three times a day plus two snacks. I think the snacks are partly to spread out the amount of food per meal. And also, it is an event. It is something consistent and pleasurable. The IOI was actually good at providing snacks.

However, since Mike had GERD and a consistent cough, the speech therapist (why do we need one of them?) prescribed (can they do that?) Thick It (which will make you gag).

Thick It makes fluids the consistency of egg whites. Mike had to have Thick It in all fluids. As if it wasn't hard enough to get him to drink fluids, now we had to make everything undrinkable. Seriously, you couldn't drink it; you squished it around in your mouth like Jell-O. Can you imagine drinking coffee like that? Let's review:

they keep him from the odds of choking to death by making life a little less worth living.

There was one thing they did that made me wonder what planet I landed on: Activities. Open any website or look at any brochure and you will quickly get to Activities with pictures of good-looking older people around a table doing something amazing. Activities are applauded by medical professionals, doctors, and highly educated experts. It is almost as if Activities will cure the residents as it improves their lives.

The IOI has an Activities Director. That's how much they believed it was important. She was a nice enough person and chatted constantly. I gave her one point for adding a person's voice to a room of zombie-like dementia residents. First, she gathered everyone around in a semicircle. I gave her another point for the interaction with each of the residents, even if some of them resented her intrusion. Her schedule was always just after lunch, which was when the rest of the staff took their lunch. So the Activities person was the only person on the floor. Now for the activity, let's say it is American Presidents' Day. Maybe one of the residents is actually cognitive enough to pay attention. The other residents:

1. Are aware she is in the room but don't know who she is (although she does look a little familiar).
2. Are aware she is in the room but don't care.
3. Are aware she is in the room and resent her constant chattering (that one would be my Mom).
4. Are aware she is in the room but would rather read the paper (that one is Mike).
5. Are aware she is in the room but would rather be back in their own room.
6. Are aware she is in the room and try to be pleasant about it.
7. Are not aware she is in the room.
8. Are not aware she is in the room and not aware they are in the room.

I have witnessed this many, many times, and I didn't come into it with any bias. I simply kept observing the blank look in all those faces. And yet the Activities person never picked up on her lack of influence.

"Now, can anyone tell me the name of our first president?" she would ask. "Anyone?"

A shaky hand from the newest resident, "Lincoln?"

"Well, Lincoln was certainly a very important president..."

How could anyone witness one of these sessions and come away with ANY reason to believe they were doing anything productive? People in the later stages of dementia do not think like us, so our normal perspective is useless:

1. We have a sense of time; they don't.
2. We have goals, plans, aspirations; they don't.
3. We sense obligation, duty, commitment; they don't.
4. We strive to be happy; they don't.
5. We have a past and a future; they don't.

For us, the present is between the past and future. For them, the present is all there is.

But I feel one thing is true: We sense, feel, harbor, and crave love. And <u>so do they</u>.

Love is not a physical need for survival. It is a spiritual need that gives us a reason to live. It is not "housed" in our brain, but more a child of our soul. Love needs to be nourished, fostered, protected, applied, practiced, encouraged, and celebrated. Once fully matured, love will endure. It even endures past death, as I can feel the love of my Mom as I write about this now. So when planning their activities, I believe they should start with love.

> Tip #13: So how do we enhance their lives on their terms? First, of course, we give up on our perspective. We stop making paper people chains.

The Activities person was doing several things right. She was physically present. And she was talking. She could have gone to each person individually, touched them softly, and looked into their blank eyes. Then told them they were loved. The stare would remain blank, but the soul would hear.

Not exactly an activity, but the facility did something else right. They set up a little nursery with baby dolls and rocking chairs. Some of the residents took to the dolls and held them lovingly. So, that worked.

They also had a great "activity" dropped in their lap. There was a girl that volunteered to come and visit the Memory Care residents about once a month. She sang to the residents using a microphone with the background music playing on a recorder. Then she would go around the room and share the microphone for the residents to join in. I witnessed a gentleman who hardly spoke at all sit up and belt out every word of *America the Beautiful*. When singing *Amazing Grace*, the girl was accompanied by a chorus of voices. Mom was one of those voices. She couldn't speak a complete sentence, but she could recite all the lyrics of several songs. According to what I have read, music is one of the last parts of the brain to be affected by Alzheimer's. You would think the activities person would have picked up on that and started a karaoke band. You would think that the whole profession of very intelligent people would have picked up on this "activity." Do I sound bitter?

Another volunteer brought in a dog. The dog was always a big hit. The facility I liked the most, but couldn't afford, had a pet in each unit. Dogs are magic. They love attention. They give love as constantly as it is accepted. Wait. They…give…love. Love, the basis of a person's existence. The enduring aspect of a person's being.

It has to be the right dog, with the right demeanor. And there are a bunch of them, waiting to be adopted. So why aren't they in Memory Care? Allergies, maybe? Maybe so, there can be a few obstacles. But the benefits are too obvious, too grand, and too important. If there is some government restriction, that government needs to be corrected.

Cats are great, too. I am a cat person. Cats more or less accept love. It is very comforting to pet a cat. A cat's purr is medicinal.

Children. My kids visited Mom with the grandkids. Mom didn't know who they were, but she enjoyed them immensely. I can't think of how to apply that on an ongoing basis.

I think a TV could be a good thing. But not TV programs. Maybe just colorful pictures of beautiful landscapes, babies, and animals. And nice background music. Mom would watch TV with Mike, but she couldn't follow the plot. She would get mad.

Personally, I would let them drink, smoke, and smoke pot. Maybe drink conservatively, but smoke all they wanted. Stop thinking we are trying to save them. Just try to give them any form of comfort. Like soft, loose-fitting clothes. Fleece sheets and covers. A soft bed. Warm clothes. A warm room. A blanket to wrap up in like a nice hug.

December 2014

Mom weighs 135 lbs. (up 2). Mike weighs 171 lbs. (up 2, will not reach this weight again)

12/21/2014 - Mike's daughter comes for a visit. It upsets Mom. Mom never liked her and used to hate visiting her with Mike. She did out of obligation, but she didn't like it. So Mom didn't know Dale, but she still knew Judy F.

January 2015

Mom weighs 132 lbs. (down 3). Mike weighs 168 lbs. (down 3)

1/9/2015 - Mom whispers so as not to be overheard. Tells us to be quiet as well. Doesn't want to attract any attention.

Urinary Tract Infection - An ailment that changes personality. Mom started having what seemed like back-to-back UTIs. Dale said that Mom infected herself by wiping back to front. The problem in fixing the problem is that first you have to test for it. You get a urine sample. You have to send the sample to the lab. Samples go out on Wednesdays. You have to pay extra to have the sample sent same day. We always asked for, and paid for, same day. The lab determines the type of bacteria, and that information has to be sent to the doctor. The doctor prescribes an antibiotic that fights that bacteria. The prescription is filled, logged, and administered. After the last pill you test for confirmation that the medicine cured the UTI. All of that would be handled by the DON. But the DON had to be asked to complete each step, and then I had to confirm that it was done. Some of the steps were close together, so you could keep track of keeping the DON on track. But you had to write down the number of days of the prescription to know when to call the DON and ask for a confirmation test. It was beyond my level of patience to keep calling the DON to ask her to do her job.

My sister took over that particular issue. She used her sweet yet firm voice to talk to the DON. She stayed on the DON and did not let anything slide. My sister was also attentive to Mom's mood swings to help determine the effectiveness of the meds.

February 2015

Mom weighs 133 lbs. (up 1). Mike weighs 167 lbs. (down 1)

March 2015

Mom weighs 131 lbs. (down 2). Mike weighs 160 lbs. (down 7)

3/8/2015 - Mom needs to be fed, but Mike is still feeding himself. We lose Delores; she went to work elsewhere. Very sad.

April 2015

Mom weighs 131 lbs. (no change). Mike weighs 165 lbs. (up 5)

4/9/2015 - Ordered a wheelchair for Mike. Worked on getting Mom's Tramadol doses right. Too much and Mom turned into a zombie. Not enough and Mom was in pain and jittery. Changed it several times and noted the changes. Dale handled that issue.

4/28/2015 - More and more Mike wanted to be fed. He could feed himself, but he just didn't want to. "If you want me to eat, you have to feed me."

Mom was at a stage where she didn't open her mouth. Sometimes it worked to place the spoon lightly on her lips. If I could get something sweet on her tongue, she would eat more. But much of the time she just clamped her mouth shut tight. Another "new reality" was that she sometimes kept her eyes closed. I don't know why she did that. Maybe it was her way of shutting out the world.

Their care level was going up, and so was the price. They had become the least capable of all the other residents, and probably the next to go. Their doctor, aware of their condition, signed for them to receive Hospice care.

PART FOUR:

A FEDERAL PROGRAM THAT WORKS

Hospice - Help when you need it the most

Hospice is an end-of-life organization tasked to provide dignity and humane treatment for the terminally ill. It also provides assistance to the family, including bereavement support after death.

May 2015

Mom weighs 138 lbs. (up 7, she will not reach this weight again). Mike weighs 163 lbs. (down 2)

5/5/2015 – I met with the Hospice nurse to register Mom and Mike into the program. His title was Clinical Liaison and his job was to coordinate with his staff, suppliers, the IOI, the doctor, and the family. His name was Charles, and he was a very busy man. He explained that he worked for AseraCare, which was a private company that provided palliative care. AseraCare was paid by Medicare under a Medicare-provider agreement.

Just like when Dale came into my life, Hospice was like the cavalry coming to the rescue (cue bugle horn, again). In addition to Charles, we got Tammy. She was a RN and would be the Case Manager assigned to us. Sarah was the aide assigned to us. Tammy and Sarah were actually angels—their wings tucked in under their scrubs. They would be with us to the end.

Finally, Dale would have someone intelligent to work with. They were on par with Dale's level of caregiving, and they partnered with Dale to improve Mom and Mike's treatment at the IOI (which Dale now referred to as the Institute of Idiots).

Charles informed me that he met with Mom and Mike. I pressed for his opinion as to how much longer they had. He had worked with many patients, and based on his experience, he predicted three months. I tried to look somber, but inside I was elated. I had been watching the cruel punishment of the disease that was eating her brain. She suffered pain, fear, infections, confusion, anxiety, anger, and all things hopeless. Death would be her escape.

I was also happy for myself. I selfishly looked forward to the release from commitment. I did not feel guilty about it. Guilt has no value.

I didn't feel the same about Mike. I didn't even like him. But, Mom had confided that her life with Mike was better than her life with Dad. Mike earned my care for his love for my Mom. We cared for him at the level that Mom would have cared for him. Privately, though, I hoped he would go first. I wanted Mom to myself at the end.

Charles explained that Hospice wasn't about living longer, it was about living better—without pain.

Sarah would come on Monday, Wednesday, and Friday mornings. She would bathe and dress Mom and Mike. So we KNEW Mom and Mike were cared for those mornings. Then she would get them to breakfast.

5/12/2015 - Mike's wheelchair comes in. We held off as long as possible because walking to meals was all the exercise Mike ever got.

5/21/2015 - Hospital beds arrive, courtesy of Hospice. I held off as long as possible on getting separate beds. But Mike was now a potential hazard to Mom. We feared he would roll over on her or try to crawl over her. Plus, hospital beds can be raised for changing or bathing, and also lowered closer to the floor. The head and feet could be raised as needed for comfort. And they could roll out of the way when necessary.

5/22/2015 - Mom leans over to the left, her head almost sideways. It is physically hard to push her up straight, as if she is using all her muscles to stay crooked. It makes it especially hard to feed her when her mouth is sideways. Also, her eyes are closed and she clenches her mouth shut.

5/23/2015 - Mom eats 75%. Mike eats 50%. He is very cranky about eating. They both get Ensure to help with nutrition.

June 2015

Mom weighs 133 lbs. (down 5). Mike weighs 157 lbs. (down 6)

6/5/2015 – I paid to have Mike's sister flown in from Georgia. Mom and Mike always enjoyed Kay's visits, so I thought they would like having her around for a week. I figured she would sit with them for most of the day, and stay with us instead of a hotel. First day, Kay was flustered by Mom and Mike's condition. Mike knew her but gave her no attention. Mom wasn't aware of anyone in the room. Kay watched us feed Mom and Mike, and then came home with us. She didn't go back. Instead, she stayed in our gazebo and chain-smoked cigarettes. She talked endlessly about working in a textile plant. And then she started repeating the same stories. We had to endure four more days of her constant storytelling. It was such a relief to get her back on a plane to go home. She said she enjoyed her visit and would like to come back someday.

Tip #14: Not all your good ideas are good ideas. But keep trying.

Mom eating close to 100% and Mike about 50% during that time.

6/12/2015 - Mike's birthday. We made him his favorite: blueberry pie. The relatives from Maine sent cookies. We are not all that concerned that Mike is diabetic; it is under control and the least of his worries.

6/15/2015 - Mom eats 100%, Mike eats 10%.

July 2015

Mom weighs 126 lbs. (down 7). Mike weighs 153 lbs. (down 4)

7/12/2015 - Unusually good day. Dale said to Mom, "I love you." Mom replied, "I love you too."

Mom ate 100%, Mike ate 50%.

7/28/2015 - Tammy reports that Mike's arm circumference dropped from 35 centimeters to 29 centimeters. That's about 13.8 inches down to 11.4 inches. He had lost that much muscle tone since they first measured him. Dale finally asks for help from the staff when feeding.

Mom ate 70%, Mike ate 20%.

August 2015

Mom weighs 126 lbs. (no change). Mike weighs 153 lbs. (no change)

8/14/2015 - Tammy reports that Mike is failing. Mark called Mike's daughter (Judy F), who plans to come the next day. Mike looks exhausted and sleeps most of the day.

8/16/2015 – Judy F gets there and feeds him at lunch and dinner. Meals are changed to puree, which makes it hard to tell what is fixed. The green stuff was beans. The white stuff was mashed potatoes. The light brown stuff was usually chicken. It all tasted like what it was. The meal was always followed up with Ensure.

8/17/2015 - Mike is feeling better. Judy F leaves to go back home.

Mom still knows Mike. They hold hands when seated next to each other. I warned Mike that someday Mom might forget who he is. Mike was not worried. "I'll just tell her it's me."

September 2015

Mom weighs 125 lbs. (down 1). Mike weighs 147 lbs. (down 6)

9/1/2015 - We are feeding them at least for lunch, sometimes lunch and dinner. We know they are getting breakfast at least three days a week and have some confidence that they are getting fed the other mornings as well. It takes all of the lunch hour to feed Mom. It requires constant prodding. She only opens her mouth a little bit at a time, so we have to be quick. Mike, on the other hand, opens wide and takes big bites. We add Ensure to every meal.

October 2015

Mom weighs 125 lbs. (no change). Mike weighs 144 lbs. (down 3)

10/1/2015 - The Hospice nurse, Tammy, visits them once a week. Mom's stats are generally good. Mike's will be fair and usually has low blood pressure.

I watch Mom and Mike and wonder what could possibly be worth living for. They are past their predicted expiration dates. I wonder if meals are the highlight of their days. For Mike, maybe it is the relief of lying down to rest.

I needed an answer. The only thing I could come up with is our inborn instinct to survive and procreate. So our reason to keep living is that life itself is precious, even if there isn't anything left to live for. Still, I wondered if we were doing them wrong by going through so much effort to keep them fed. Maybe their lack of appetite was in concert with their rate of decline. Maybe we were just prolonging their misery.

November 2015

Mom weighs 119 lbs. (down 6). Mike weighs 141 lbs. (down 3)

December 2015

Mom weighs 122 lbs. (up 3). Mike weighs 140 lbs. (down 1)

12/14/2015 - Dale purchased eight pairs of socks for Mike and six pairs of slacks with elastic waistbands for Mom. She also bought a set of sheets and more towels. It angers Dale that laundry is lost, but I shrug it off.

For some reason staff keeps putting a bra on Mom. Dale finds all the bras and throws them away.

Hospice reports that their weights are dropping a lot, but Mom's heart remains strong. This gives me hope that she will outlive Mike.

12/25/2015 - Dale's daughter and family are sailing in the Bahamas. They have a daughter and a son. Dale's son and his wife also have a daughter and son. Dale's son put together a trip to have them and us go to the Bahamas for Christmas. We had Christmas early with my kids, then flew to Exuma. It was my first non-traditional Christmas, and hopefully not my last. I thought about Mom and Mike, but I was distracted by warm breezes. And I relearned something: a caregiver needs to take a break now and then.

> Tip #15: Take a break. It will help you be a better caregiver.

January 2016

Mom weighs 122 lbs. (no change). Mike weighs 135 lbs. (down 5)

1/10/2016 - Dale continues her fight with the DON and IOI. She will not give up trying to improve the living conditions. Staff has wipes on hand to clean residents' hands but doesn't use them. The toilet broke and went unfixed. It was full of poop. Mom and Mike were wearing the same clothes from the day before. Their bedding consisted of a thin, wrinkled sheet over a plastic mattress. The skin on Mike's butt has started to break down. It is red, raw, and really sore to the touch. Same for Mom. This is a report card for their level of care. I think that having Hospice in there gave the IOI staff the impression that they didn't have to do anything.

> Tip #16: Check your modesty at the front door. Get in there and do what needs to be done. It's no different than checking a toddler's diaper.

As if the DON wasn't useless enough, she started to make things worse. You can't restrain a resident. Full-length bed rails are considered restraint. Mom and Mike had been in hospital beds since last May. So they had full-length rails, which still didn't stop Mike from falling out of bed. But the DON was determined that the full rails had to be lowered. Not to worry, a floor pad would be placed between the beds at night. Yes, the DON was that stupid.

The pads were a bit of a trip hazard. The night shift pushed them under the beds.

February 2016

Mom weighs 122 lbs (no change). Mike weighs 133 lbs. (down 2)

At 122, Mom's weight was only four pounds less than three years before. However, at 133, Mike had lost 51 pounds over those three years. And he was the better eater.

2/1/2016 - I remodel kitchens for a living. Work comes in spurts. On that day I started a remodeling project.

The DON thinks the beds should be separated. I take my concerns to the manager. He concurs with the DON's opinion. Stupid.

PART FIVE:

TAKING BACK CONTROL

FINALLY! FOR THE FIRST, ONLY, AND MOST CRITICAL TIME, I GET AHEAD OF THE NEW REALITY!

2/2/2016 - I get home from work and I am bushed. I am too late to go to the IOI. I take a shower and Dale has a (as usual) delicious dinner waiting. I am off vodka but not wine, which goes oh so good with lasagna.

Dale informs me that the manager won't budge on the bed issue. It is getting late, about 8 PM, and I decide to go and have a look for myself. Entering their room as quietly as possible, I find Mike asleep in his bed, which is pushed up against the wall. Mom's bed is pushed up against his bed, with her rail up and the floor pad next to the bed. For once I was grateful that the DON rarely communicated anything to her staff. The night shift had pushed the beds together and pulled the full rail up, probably because it made sense.

They were facing the far wall, so I was behind them when I turned to leave. Mom made a sound of some sort and I was afraid I had woken her up. I went over to the side of her bed just to check. Her eyes were closed, as they always were, but she did make a sound. And then she raised her arm up toward me. It was as if she were saying, "Help me! Save me!" I took her hand and held it to my chest. The room was quiet and dark, and I realized that if I had not been there at that moment, her outstretched hand would have gone unseen. My heart ripped in half. Tears made everything blurry. I rushed out and into my truck and drove home. All the headlights looked like starbursts.

Dale was watching TV. When I walked in and stood in front of the TV, she could see that something was very wrong. She probably thought I was going to tell her that one of them had died. She turned off the TV. I got on my knees and put my head on her lap and sobbed. I slowed down long enough to say Mom and Mike were okay. Then I cried again uncontrollably.

There was no way we could bring them home; we had been over that time and again. It wasn't an option. But I make all important decisions with my heart, not my head.

I stopped crying long enough to say, "Dale, I need to bring my Mom home to die!" And then I started crying again. When I finally slowed down to a whimper she cupped my cheeks in her hands and smiled. "Duh," she said, "What took you so long?"

Between Mark, Judy, and I, all important decisions were determined by the majority. We were almost always unanimous. I was going to bring Mom home but called them for their approval. My sister said, "Yes, if that is what you want." And my brother said, "Yes, if you think we can swing it. You're taking on a big responsibility."

2/3/2016 - I gave notice verbally, then faxed it in writing. The manager actually asked me, "What made you decide to do this?"

Because you're an idiot! I can't take you abusing them anymore! I wouldn't leave my dog there! You're a joke! Inept! Incompetent!

I did not verbalize my thoughts. I simply said, "It's time," and hung up.

I had to go to work. In my absence, Dale sprung into action. She had been wanting them home for a long time. She hated the IOI. By the time I got home, she had emptied one of my office bookcases and dragged it into the dining room. That is where we would put them. The bookcase was fully stocked with diapers, wipes, gloves, lotions, clothes (new), washcloths, towels, a dish pail, cans of Ensure, puddings, and some baby food. I was amazed but not surprised. She is the ultimate caregiver.

"We need to find a place for the table and chairs," she said.

"What happened to the stuff on my bookcase?" I asked.

"What stuff?"

There was so much to do. Hospice would follow us home, of course. We would get Sarah FIVE times a week and Tammy would check in a few times a week. They both knew us by now and were very supportive of our decision. Charles would order beds and supplies. Hospice provided bed pads, gloves, bed tables, body soaps, and diapers.

My sister took the dining room table and chairs.

We needed a baby monitor, a food processor, a pill crusher, a blood pressure monitor, and an oxygen monitor.

Dale bought all things soft: flannel pajamas, flannel sheets, fleece blankets, extra pillows.

Mark jumped in on getting things out of IOI as much as possible. Some things had to stay, but much of it was just in the way. None of it came to our house.

Also needed were the medications, which included morphine (thanks to Hospice). Pain would be prevented.

Meanwhile, the IOI went into hyperstupidity. Mike was still sliding out of bed, given the lack of using the bed rails. The director informed me that they decided to put them in separate rooms: Mom in the living area and Mike back in the bedroom. Their "reasoning" was, out of sight, out of mind. Mike would not get out of bed. Really?

That night, Mike got out of bed. He must have gained some momentum before doing a face plant on the carpet. His face was a mess, and there was a rug burn on his shoulder. That injury would not heal before he died.

I was still on my business project, so Dale did most of the work. We could have gotten Mom and Mike home by February 12, but only one of the beds came in. The supplier didn't see the quantity of "2." The other bed was reordered, but that took us into the weekend. We couldn't bring Mom and Mike home until we had both beds. Charles promised the bed on February 15, and he also coordinated with the IOI and the company that could transport wheelchairs. He scheduled them on that date as well, which made me a little nervous.

It was a very cold day, and that made me concerned about Mom and Mike staying warm. I was pacing back and forth and saw a van backing into our driveway. I yelled to Dale, "The bed is here!" She was in the laundry room.

Then I saw the driver open the side door and I was shocked to see wheelchairs.

"Dale! It's Mom and Mike!"

We rushed out to help the driver get them out of the van and into the house. I was livid. The Institute of Idiots sent two souls out into the cold two hours early with no communication with us. And the transport company was none the wiser.

Charles was just as angry. "I will have a bed there within the hour," he said. He called the supplier and got their commitment to get the bed to us. Then he called to tell us, and then called later to confirm we got it. He did not like it when suppliers let him down.

We got Mom and Mike out of their clothes, bathed them, and put them in flannel pajamas. We laid them on flannel sheets and covered them with fleece blankets. Then we fed them. We served warm, pureed chicken covered in gravy. We gave them pureed potato salad, and pureed green beans. Then real ice cream, and coffee from the Keurig. They ate it all.

Then, life got complicated. Meds had to be organized, crushed first, then added to pudding. We used shot glasses to mix the meds with the pudding. Meals were prepared in advance. The blender stayed on the countertop next to the sink. Feeding and changing them filled the day. We also had to feed ourselves and organize our own meds. We had two cats and a dog, so that was a few more meals, plus litter boxes. And Dale's daughter was still in the Bahamas, so we had her three cats as well. The cats didn't get along, so we had to keep them separated. We had to deal with five litter boxes plus messy adult briefs.

Tools and things that helped

Dale bought a dish rack. I don't know how she knew that doing the dishes was no longer a matter of running the dishwasher when full. It was more dynamic than that. We used the plates with three sections. We only had a few, so they had to be washed after each meal. Spoons were plastic and got washed by hand. Plastic is softer than metal and easier on their lips. Since meds were mixed with pudding in shot glasses, they had to be washed constantly. The food processor parts lived in the dish rack.

The food processor was a beast. It is not a blender. A blender is for making margaritas. A food processor is a whole different thing. It takes anything and turns it to puree. Sometimes it needed some liquid, but not much. Sometimes we added gravy instead of just water.

The baby monitor was a useful tool. It had a screen that somehow worked in the dark. You could tell if Mom and Mike were still or moving. It was also portable. The camera stayed on the bookcase and the monitor came with us. It was next to my bed at night, in the kitchen most of the day, and under the TV when we were in the den. Surprisingly, the audio portion was the most useful feature. A new sound told you when to look at the screen. And at night, I could turn up the volume a bit and hear Mom's breathing (which was louder than Mike's). Toward the end, her breathing became shallow.

We have a dog named Puppy. Mike called him Trixie. That was the name of Mom's dog, back when Mom and Mike met. Mike was always delighted when Puppy came into the room.

We bought a second cable box and set up a TV for Mike to watch *Gunsmoke* reruns. That and *Andy Griffith*. I couldn't stop watching them when feeding Mom or Mike. Those shows are wonderfully simple and well written. Mike was sometimes alert enough to watch TV, or at least we thought he was. We never did figure him out.

Still, we were in over our heads. We needed help. I put an ad in Craigslist. I got about thirty responses right away and more came in every day. You could tell some of them were form letters:

Dear Sir/Madam: I am writing in response to your ad for a position in your company. Attached is my resume.

Those were easy to cast aside. I called some that were anywhere near normal. And that eliminated more. Most didn't understand that we just wanted someone for a few hours now and then. We finally found a lady that lived close by, didn't have a job to go to, and would work for us as much or as little as we wanted. Her name was Ann.

February 20 & 21, 2016 (Saturday and Sunday) - Had the new lady, Ann, over from 7:30 AM to 10 AM. It was nice to have help with the meds, feeding, changing, and bathing. After we finished a meal and cleaned up, it was almost time to prepare for the next meal.

Tip #17: Pull in the help, as much as you can afford.

The rest of February 2016 - We had Mom home, safe. But we didn't have her awake. Her eyes never opened, and her most common communication was a groan when we moved her from side to side. That wasn't enough for Dale. She would slip into bed with Mom and hold her. She had her phone, and would pull up Alison

Krauss singing *Down To The River To Pray*. She played it over and over. I think Mom knew she was home and could finally let go.

Mom forgot who I was months before. And complete sentences were a thing of the past. Sitting next to her, I didn't expect conversation. But then she mumbled a few last words:

"I traded you for a dog," she said.

"Get a good deal?" I asked.

"Uh-huh."

Then later, her final words spoken to me: "Jesus didn't call back." My only guess is that she was waiting for Him to take her Home.

3/1/2016 - Dale informed me of the next reality, which would be the last reality. Mom had stopped eating and her body was shutting down. There was no more than two weeks left.

It hit me like a ton of bricks. Mom's death was always off in the future; the present was for dealing with all the challenges. Now her death was in the present. I was actually surprised. It felt as if

Mom kept dying over and over again, a little at a time.

I had work commitments. I did as much as I could to finish some tasks, but my heart wasn't in it. I got Mom this far, and I wanted to be there at the end.

But Mom was in good hands. Dale held her and played *Down To The River To Pray* over and over. It was their song.

Dale was passionate that Mom not be in pain. Under Tammy's direction as to dosage, Dale gave morphine when needed. Mom could not speak, but we knew when she was hurting. Her furled brow was one of the indicators. Dale kept her brow relaxed.

Dale was also passionate about their skin condition. A diaper rash was unacceptable. It was a common problem at the IOI, but not on Dale's watch. She kept them changed, clean, and lathered with lotion.

I was amazed at all the diapers we went through. We literally filled the trash container. I was also amazed that Dale could change people heavier than her. She rolled them over by pulling an arm and hip, and the body eventually followed. She rolled her side of the diaper in on itself. She wiped and lathered that half of their butt. Then a new diaper was tucked in between the old diaper and skin. Somehow, when she rolled them over the other way, the old diaper was underneath the new diaper and she pulled it out without a problem. That's how she did it. When I did it by myself, I got poop all over the new diaper, the chuck (bed liner), and sometimes the bedding.

On one occasion in particular, I got up in the middle of the night to check on them, and Mike was a mess. Changing his diaper was such a disaster that I ended up changing his pajamas and bedding. I was so tired and sleepy. I could have used Dale's help. But she needed a break as much and as often as possible. I let her sleep.

Dale's weight after three weeks: 110 lbs. (down 6)

March 8, 2016 5:20 PM

Dale called around noon and said it was time to come home. I had just finished up and was already on the road.

My brother and sister were already there when I arrived. There wasn't much conversation. We were there together sharing a tender family moment.

Dale had rolled Mom's bed from the dining room and into the living room. It was the room I used as my office and it had enough room for the bed. Mike wasn't all that aware of what was going on around him, but Dale didn't want to take any chances. Mike just slept.

We had no idea how long we would be waiting, not that it mattered. Mark had reports to turn in, so he left. He said to just call him when something happened.

Then we started a list of people to call, and a list of information needed for the obituary. Judy was on my computer looking up examples.

I stood on Mom's right side and Dale was seated on the bed on her left. The rails were down; they were no longer needed. My sister was sitting at my desk and reading some of the things we would need to know. It helped to have something productive to do. We were in no hurry, and at one point, Judy was staring at the screen but not saying anything. That helped put the room in a more reverent mode.

"She's gone," said Dale.

It registered slowly. I looked down. Dale was holding Mom's hand and looking closely at her face. She placed her other hand on Mom's chest for a moment.

Mom was gone. Jesus had called back.

A natural silence fell as we each dealt with our thoughts and emotions. Judy quickly called Mark. I didn't feel too much. Just numbness. But I was grateful that I was there. And grateful that Mom no longer suffered the fear and confusion—the abuse, really.

I was grateful that we weren't at the IOI with regulations that we couldn't do something or *had* to do something. Our sacred moment wasn't under the control of heartless idiots. We had Mom to ourselves, and we reported to no one (until we were ready). She was home—with us.

And I was grateful for Dale.

When Mark arrived, we talked about different things. Mostly we shared our loss without the intervention of others.

When the time came, Dale called Hospice. It was after 5 PM and Tammy wasn't there. Another nurse came instead. She was pleasant and professional, but it would have been nicer to have Tammy.

The nurse called the funeral home; all of that information was on file. Then she methodically collected and disposed of all of Mom's leftover meds.

The young assistants from the funeral home that came for Mom were very professional, courteous, and respectful. I was impressed.

Mark had to leave, but Judy stayed. Dale's son brought over dinner. That was timely.

Then Dale sat on the edge of Mike's bed and talked to him. She explained that Mom had died. I stood off to the side, watching. Mike got very upset and starting crying. She asked him if he knew why he was upset. Mike said, "Yes," and pointed to me. "Because I don't know how I'm going to pay this guy!"

He settled down after a while. He didn't ask about Mom, so we were grateful that the dementia kept him from suffering as much.

> Tip #18: As of this writing, there is no cure for Alzheimer's.

3/9/2016 - More luck: Mom had everything planned and paid for

Both Mom and Mike had planned and paid for their funeral and burial. So all we had to do was pick out the flowers. I assumed we would be coddled and handled delicately as we were guided through the process. That's the way it looks when you're visiting a funeral for someone else. The guys in suits are always so helpful. Our Funeral Director, however, had more of a "it will all work out" attitude. Had this funeral been more emotional, his treatment would have been considered negligent.

There were people that came and expressed condolences, but for me it just seemed like something to get done and over with.

Because of too much rain, Mom couldn't be buried on the day of the funeral. So on the following day a service was held in the mausoleum. It was on a

Monday, so only family came. Instead of a service, we each got up and talked about a memory of her. As we were leaving I turned around and looked back at Mom's casket. She was left at the far end, and we were all leaving out the door. It felt wrong to just leave her there, by herself. I had gotten her this far but fell short of having her buried. I had to snap out of it and leave. It was done. Finished. The end.

I few days later we went to the cemetery and checked her gravesite. The dirt mound had already started to settle. She was laid to rest next to Dad.

Mike is still with us...

I didn't wish him any harm, but there was no longer a direct tie to me as family. It was more of an obligation to care for him. His care would not be based on who he was; it would be based on who we were. So we just went back into caregiver mode.

I never saw a difference between Mom's Alzheimer's and Mike's dementia. His decline was very similar to Mom's and, remarkably, at the same pace. Even though Hospice predicted his demise at the same time, I figured he would last for a year or more. He was tough and never complained. He never said he was in pain, even though it was obvious. So looking ahead to the summer, I didn't make any plans.

Our house smelled like a latrine. Mike pooped continuously. The smell was "in my nose" even when out at the grocery store or somewhere. If this story is about advice regarding caregiving, it is now about caring for a non-relative that you don't even like. It is harder and less rewarding. More like work.

On that note, there is an aspect of caregiving that didn't occur to me until it was all over. And that is the pride of stepping up to the challenge.

There are situations where I am asked, "Military?" My answer is no. I did not serve. I did nothing to protect our country's freedom. I was eligible at the end of Vietnam, had a high lottery number, and didn't enlist. That is not "a feather in my cap."

However, on a different but equal level, I served as a caregiver. In all my life, it is probably the biggest "feather in my cap." I raised a family, but that had more joy than effort. I finished college. But there isn't anything in my life that equals the title of caregiver. It gives me pride, and I am passing it along as a tip.

Tip #19: Judge all the other things that keep you busy with the importance of caring for another soul. The amount of effort it requires is equal to the personal reward it brings.

Mom's Death Certificate

The funeral home called and Mom's Death Certificate was ready. I picked it up and looked it over. The cause of her death was Cardiopulmonary Arrest, which means her heart stopped.

Below that, under "Other significant conditions contributing to death but not resulting in the underlying cause given in Part I," was diabetes. Mom didn't have diabetes; Mike had diabetes. Someone pulled the wrong file.

You wouldn't think there could be errors on a Death Certificate under any circumstances. But there is no crosschecking. Administrative personnel don't know anything about the deceased.

Mike follows Mom…

It seemed like a long time having Mike. In reality, it was only a month. In that time, he mostly slept. He didn't seem to wake up while getting a bath or getting changed.

April 13, 2016 - Tammy and Dale agreed that Mike was very close. We had been in touch with his daughter, so she was on her way that day. She arrived at 7 PM and sat with her Dad. She wanted to stay all night, but she was too tired. We promised to stay with Mike and let her know as soon as anything changed. She left to go check into a hotel.

Dale went to bed. I stayed up with Mike. His breathing was so shallow there were several times I thought he had died.

At 3 AM, Dale got up to relieve me. I was grateful to go to bed. I slept until 6:30 AM. I was tired but too awake to stay in bed. I got up and fixed coffee, and Dale was sitting next to Mike. We talked about calling his daughter, but it was hard to judge the timing. It could be soon or another day or more. So we left it up to her as to when she would return.

At 7:15 AM, I left the room to get a second cup of coffee. From the other room Dale announced, "He's gone."

Just like that. One minute a barely living person, and the next minute, gone. In a way, his death gave closure to Mom's death. It was now all over.

We called Mike's daughter. She came quickly and sat with him for some time. She cried again and again. When the time came, we called Hospice and the same nurse arrived. She pronounced Mike's death, then methodically disposed of all of his remaining meds.

Same funeral home, same cemetery

Having just been through the ceremony, we guided Mike's daughter through the viewings, funeral, and cemetery. Her family came; all of them were from out of town. It was very awkward.

As with Mom, there had been too much rain to bury Mike on the day of the funeral. So the service was held in the mausoleum. I had arranged to have Army representatives there. Two of them came. They ceremoniously lifted the flag off the casket, folded it, and presented it to Mike's daughter. She kept thanking us, but we just wanted to get away.

PART SIX:

RECOVERY FOR THE CAREGIVER

A time of renewal

Our next new reality was total normalcy. First, we couldn't wait to get the hospital bed, wheelchairs, bedside potty, bedside pad, and everything associated with caregiving out of the house. Then Dale cleaned the house fanatically. She moved my office into the dining room, where Mom and Mike had been. She moved the dining room into the family room, which was brilliant. It provided much more space around the chairs. The family room furniture went to the living room, which is at the front of the house.

During that time we went shopping for a new sofa. My old sofa was disgusting. We looked at several, and Dale picked one to buy. I was a little surprised. I had not seen her buy anything for herself since I met her. Her favorite clothing store is Goodwill. And she only buys things on sale. But I think in this case, she knew she deserved it. She needed our home to be reborn. Later, she gave a nod to a new coffee table. It was expensive and not on sale. Add To Cart.

Pictures were moved around. I built a TV cabinet to fit exactly in the space she picked. She bought things to decorate each room. We were very happy with the changes. It helped put some distance between us and Alzheimer's.

> Tip #20: Get on with your life, change your surroundings, and reward yourself for having taken on a huge responsibility.

They just keep on dying...

Mail kept coming in for both of them. Mostly for Mike, and mostly from charitable causes. He must have donated to a lot of places. He got more mail than I did. For mail that had a postage-paid return envelope, I wrote "deceased" and sent it back. Many of them kept coming back anyway. He received notice that his medical benefits would end after one year. I tossed that one. Magazine subscriptions kept coming in. I am still getting medical bills.

Oddly, there is a track on the porch from one of the wheelchairs that brought Mom and Mike home. It is black and won't fade away.

I sometimes think of Mom when I put the silverware away. When I moved into the house, Mom took the task of organizing the knives and spoons and forks. They are still in the same trays she put them in. It puts a lump in my throat.

The following May, for the first time in my life, I did not have a mother on Mother's Day.

Mom's upcoming birthday will not add another year to her age. Both of them stopped at 86. The upcoming anniversary of her death will start a new numbering sequence. We will count one…two…three years since she died. There are no pleasant memories of her decline.

If I knew then what I know now…

In the beginning of my journey, I didn't even know Mom had Alzheimer's and was going to die. All I knew was that there was a pill left in the Monday lunch slot when I checked on Tuesday. From there, I just kept reacting to new levels of decline. If only I had known what was coming, I would have been better prepared.

Looking back, I feel I could have done better. I would have kept them at home as long as possible, somehow. Even if it meant having to leave them alone sometimes, which would not be safe. Maybe I should have moved in with them. The first stages of decline only require meals, meds, and finding what they constantly misplace. And love.

In the middle stages of decline they become incontinent, need to be showered, and supervised more closely. Most of us are not able to handle that level of care. So the question is, at what point do we have to put our own needs first and let them enter outside facilities? It is a hard choice to make, and everyone's reality is different.

Let love be your yardstick.

HELPFUL RESOURCES

For more information about elder abuse and where to get help:

Eldercare Locator
1-800-677-1116
www.eldercare.gov

Family Caregiver Alliance
1-800-445-8106 (toll-free)
info@caregiver.org (email)
www.caregiver.org

National Adult Protective Services Association
1-217-523-4431
www.napsa-now.org

National Center on Elder Abuse
1-855-500-3537 (toll-free)
ncea@med.usc.edu (email)
www.ncea.aoa.gov

National Committee for the Prevention of Elder Abuse
1-202-464-9481

info@preventelderabuse.org (email)
www.preventelderabuse.org/elderabuse

National Domestic Violence Hotline
1-800-799-7233 (toll-free, 24/7)
1-800-787-3224 (TTY/toll-free)
www.thehotline.org/get-help

National Family Caregiver Support Program
Administration on Aging
1-202-619-0724
aclinfo@acl.hhs.gov (email)
*www.aoa.acl.gov/AoA_Programs/HCLTC/
Caregiver*

**National Library of Medicine MedlinePlus:
Elder Abuse**
www.nlm.nih.gov/medlineplus/elderabuse.html

**National Long-Term Care Ombudsman
Resource Center**
1-202-332-2275
info@theconsumervoice.org (email)
www.ltcombudsman.org

Stop Medicare Fraud: Prevent Fraud
www.stopmedicarefraud.gov/preventfraud

U.S. Department of Justice
1-202-514-2000
elder.justice@usdoj.gov (email)
www.justice.gov/elderjustice

WellSpouse® Association
1-800-838-0879 (toll-free)
info@wellspouse.org (email)
www.wellspouse.org

For information on health and aging, including resources on caregiving and Alzheimer's disease, contact:

National Institute on Aging Information Center
P.O. Box 8057
Gaithersburg, MD 20898-8057
1-800-222-2225 (toll-free)
1-800-222-4225 (toll-free/TTY)
niaic@nia.nih.gov (email)
www.nia.nih.gov
www.nia.nih.gov/espanol

Sign up for regular email alerts about new publications and find other information from the NIA.

Visit *www.nihseniorhealth.gov*, a senior-friendly website from the National Institute on Aging and the National Library of Medicine. This website has health and wellness information for older adults. Special features make it simple to use. For example, you can click on a button to make the type larger.